Dash Diet Slow Cooker Snack and Appetizers Cookbook

Creative and Tasty Recipes for your Diet

Carmela Rojas

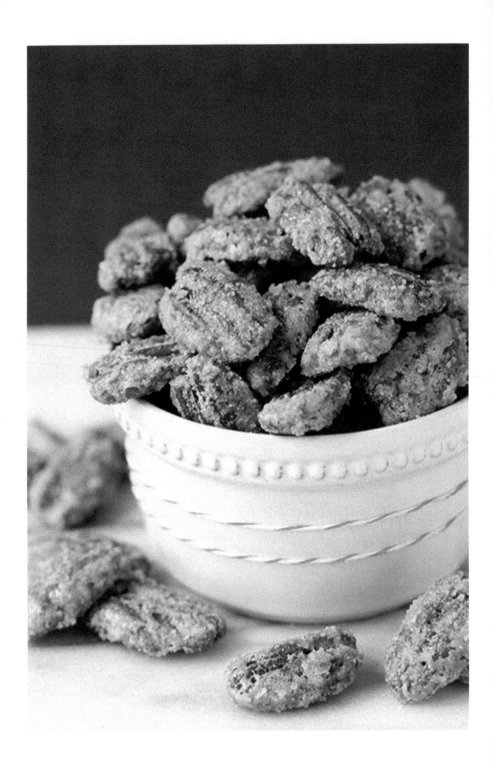

TABLE OF CONTENTS

CLAMS BOWL 6

SESAME DIP 8

SUGARED PECANS 10

CAYENNE PEPPER SPREAD 12

SPICED NUTS 14

LIME JUICE SNACK 16

GREEN ONIONS AND CORN SPREAD 18

SMOKED PAPRIKA CAULIFLOWER SPREAD 19

RICOTTA ZUCCHINI ROLLS..21

LEMON SALMON BITES...24

AMERICAN FONDUE 26

CREAM CHEESE AND KALE DIP...28

BUTTERSCOTCH DIP...30

BEER BARBECUED MEATBALLS 31

SWEET AND SPICY NUTS...34

SOUR CREAM DIP 36

HOT CRAB DIP 37

HERBED ZUCCHINI SALAD...38

ASIAN CHICKEN WINGS 40

CRANBERRIES SALAD..43

CHERRY TOMATOES AND SPINACH SALSA 45

SALMON APPETIZER MIX...47

BEET AND BASIL SPREAD 49

MEXICAN DIP..51

CREAMY SPINACH DIP 53

CREAMY MEXICAN BEEF AND BEAN DIP 54

BASIL PECANS...56

4

DILL MEAT ROLLS...58

SRIRACHA DIP...60

WALNUTS AND SEEDS BOWL..62

HOT CHEESY CRABMEAT DIP..63

SWEET AND SPICY BRATWURST..65

SWEET AND SOUR CHICKEN WINGS.....................................67

GARLIC AND TOMATO APPETIZER...70

OREGANO SALSA..72

COCKTAIL MEATBALLS...73

CREAM CHEESE DIP...75

HONEY CHICKEN WINGS...76

SALMON AND CHERRY TOMATOES SALAD.............................78

NUTMEG ENDIVE SALAD...80

SALMON AND SHALLOT SALAD..82

PEPPERCORNS ASPARAGUS...84

BROCCOLI DIP..86

CREOLE SHRIMPS..88

PARMESAN STUFFED MUSHROOMS......................................89

CINNAMON NUTS MIX..91

ALMOND FLOUR STICKS..93

SOY SAUCE CHICKEN WINGS...95

3-INGREDIENTS SHRIMP SALAD...97

STEVIA AND BULGUR SALAD..99

4-WEEK MEAL PLAN...101

5

Clams Bowl

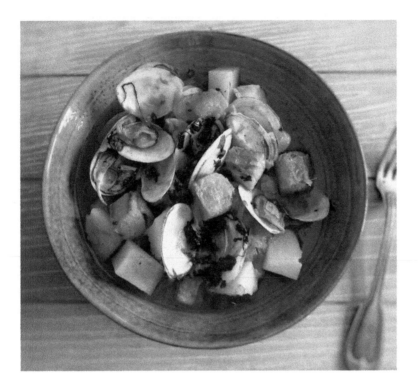

Servings: 4

Cooking Time: 2 Hours

Ingredients:

- 10 ounces low sodium veggie stock
- 40 small clams
- Lemon wedges for serving
- 1 yellow onion, chopped
- 2 tablespoons parsley, chopped

- 1 teaspoon olive oil

Directions:

1. Grease your slow cooker with the oil; add onion, clams, stock and parsley, toss, cover and cook on High for 2 hours.
2. Divide into small bowls and serve with lemon wedges on the side.

Nutrition Info:

Calories 172, Fat 1.8g, Cholesterol 0mg, Sodium 1137mg, Carbohydrate 36.5g, Fiber 1.9g, Sugars 11.5g, Protein 2.2g, Potassium 322mg

Sesame Dip

Servings: 4

Cooking Time: 2 Hours

Ingredients:
- 4 cups zucchinis, chopped
- 1 cup low-sodium chicken stock
- 4 garlic cloves, minced
- ¾ cup sesame paste
- ¼ cup olive oil
- ½ cup lemon juice
- Black pepper to the taste

Directions:
1. In your slow cooker, mix the zucchinis with stock and pepper, cover, cook on High for 2 hours, transfer to your blender, add oil, garlic, lemon juice and sesame paste, blend, divide into small bowls and serve.

Nutrition Info:

Calories 425, Fat 37.7g, Cholesterol 0mg, Sodium 99mg, Carbohydrate 17.6g, Fiber 4.1g, Sugars 3g, Protein 10.8g, Potassium 625mg

Sugared Pecans

Servings: 24 Servings

Ingredients:

- 1 pound (455 g) pecan halves
- ¼ cup (55 g) unsalted butter, melted
- ½ cup (63 g) powdered sugar
- ¼ teaspoon ground cloves
- 1½ teaspoons ground cinnamon
- ¼ teaspoon ground ginger

Directions:

1. Turn slow cooker to high for about 15 minutes. In hot slow cooker, stir together the nuts and butter. Add the powdered sugar, stirring to blend and coat evenly. Cover and cook on high for 15 minutes. Reduce the heat to low and remove lid; cook, uncovered, stirring occasionally, for about 2 to 3 hours or until the nuts are coated with a crisp glaze. Transfer the nuts to a bowl. In another small bowl, combine the spices; sift over the nuts, stirring to coat evenly. Let cool before serving.

Nutrition Info:

Per serving: 1 g water; 158 calories (83% from fat, 4% from protein, 12% from carb); 2 g protein; 16 g total fat; 2 g saturated fat; 8 g monounsaturated fat; 4 g polyunsaturated fat; 5 g carb; 2 g fiber; 3 g sugar; 53 mg phosphorus; 16 mg calcium; 1 mg iron; 0 mg sodium; 79 mg potassium; 70 IU vitamin A; 16 mg ATE vitamin E; 0 mg vitamin C; 5 mg cholesterol

Cayenne Pepper Spread

Servings: 5

Cooking Time: 5 Hours

Ingredients:
- 3 cups water
- 1 and ½ cups black-eyed peas
- ½ cup pecans, toasted
- ½ teaspoon garlic powder
- ½ teaspoon cayenne powder
- ½ teaspoon chili powder
- 1 teaspoon Cajun seasoning
- A pinch of black pepper

Directions:
1. In your slow cooker, mix the peas with Cajun seasoning, pepper and water, stir, cover and cook on High for 5 hours.
2. Drain, transfer to a blender, add pecans, garlic powder, chili powder and cayenne powder, pulse well, divide into bowls and serve as a snack

Nutrition Info:

Calories 98, Fat 4.9g, Cholesterol 0mg, Sodium 32mg, Carbohydrate 10.9g, Fiber 3.2g, Sugars 0.3g, Protein 4.3g, Potassium 164mg

Spiced Nuts

Servings: 32 Servings

Ingredients:

- ½ pound (255 g) pecan halves
- ½ pound (255 g) unsalted cashews
- ¼ cup (55 g) unsalted butter, melted
- 1 tablespoon (7.5 g) chili powder
- 1 teaspoon dried basil
- 1 teaspoon dried oregano
- 1 teaspoon dried thyme
- ½ teaspoon onion powder
- ¼ teaspoon garlic powder
- ¼ teaspoon cayenne

Directions:

1. Combine all ingredients in slow cooker. Cover and cook on high for 15 minutes. Turn to low and continue to cook, uncovered, stirring occasionally for 2 hours. Transfer nuts to a baking sheet and cool completely.

Nutrition Info:

Per serving: 1 g water; 104 calories (81% from fat, 7% from protein, 13% from carb); 2 g protein; 10 g total fat; 2 g saturated fat; 5 g monounsaturated fat; 2 g polyunsaturated fat; 4 g carb; 1 g fiber; 1 g sugar; 56 mg phosphorus; 11 mg calcium; 1 mg iron; 4 mg sodium; 76 mg potassium; 129 IU vitamin A; 12 mg ATE vitamin E; 0 mg vitamin C; 4 mg cholesterol

Lime Juice Snack

Servings: 8

Cooking Time: 2 Hours

Ingredients:
- 1 pineapple, peeled and cut into medium sticks
- 2 tablespoons stevia
- 1 tablespoon olive oil
- 1 tablespoon lime juice
- 1 tablespoon lime zest, grated
- 1 teaspoon cinnamon powder
- ¼ teaspoon cloves, ground

Directions:
1. In a bowl, mix lime juice with stevia, oil, cinnamon and cloves and whisk well.
2. Add the pineapple sticks to your slow cooker, add lime mix, toss, cover and cook on High for 2 hours.
3. Serve the pineapple sticks as a snack with lime zest sprinkled on top.

Nutrition Info:

Calories 26, Fat 1.8g, Cholesterol 0mg, Sodium 1mg, Carbohydrate 6.1 g, Fiber 0.4g, Sugars 2.1g, Protein 0.1g, Potassium 26mg

Green Onions and Corn Spread

Servings: 8

Cooking Time: 2 Hours

Ingredients:

- 8 ounces low-fat cream cheese
- 30 ounces canned corn, no-salt-added, drained
- 2 green onions, chopped
- ½ cup coconut cream
- ½ teaspoon chili powder
- 1 jalapeno, chopped

Directions:

1. In your slow cooker, mix corn with green onions, coconut cream, cream cheese, chili powder and jalapeno, cover, cook on Low for 2 hours, whisk well, divide into bowls and serve as a dip.

Nutrition Info:

Calories 631, Fat 20.3g, Cholesterol 31mg, Sodium 175mg, Carbohydrate 110.8g, Fiber 16.3g, Sugars 19.5g, Protein 21.3g, Potassium 1650mg

Smoked Paprika Cauliflower Spread

Servings: 4

Cooking Time: 7 Hours

Ingredients:
- 2 cups cauliflower florets
- 1 cup coconut milk
- 1/3 cup cashews, chopped
- 2 and ½ cups water
- 1 cup turnips, chopped
- 1 teaspoon garlic powder
- ¼ teaspoon smoked paprika
- ¼ teaspoon mustard powder

Directions:
1. In your slow cooker, mix cauliflower with cashews, turnips and water, stir, cover, cook on Low for 7 hours, drain, transfer to a blender, add milk, garlic powder, paprika and mustard powder, blend well, divide into bowls and serve as a snack

Nutrition Info:

Calories 228, Fat 19.7g, Cholesterol 0mg, Sodium 51mg, Carbohydrate 12.4g, Fiber 3.6g, Sugars 5.2g, Protein 4.6g, Potassium 445mg

Ricotta Zucchini Rolls

Servings: 24

Cooking Time: 1 Hour

Ingredients:

- 2 tablespoons olive oil
- 24 basil leaves
- 3 zucchinis, thinly sliced
- ½ cup tomato sauce, no-salt-added
- ¼ cup basil leaves, whole
- 2 tablespoons mint, chopped
- 1 and ½ cup low-fat ricotta cheese
- Black pepper to the taste

Directions:

1. Brush zucchini slices with half of the olive oil, season with the pepper and place them on a working surface.
2. In a bowl, mix ricotta with chopped basil, mint and pepper, stir well, spread this over zucchini, divide whole basil leaves, roll them, transfer to your slow cooker add the rest of the oil and the tomato sauce, cover, cook on High for 1 hour, arrange them on a platter and serve.

21

Nutrition Info:

Calories 41, Fat 2.6g, Cholesterol 5mg, Sodium 56mg, Carbohydrate 2.9g, Fiber 1g, Sugars 0.8g, Protein 2.4g, Potassium 152mg

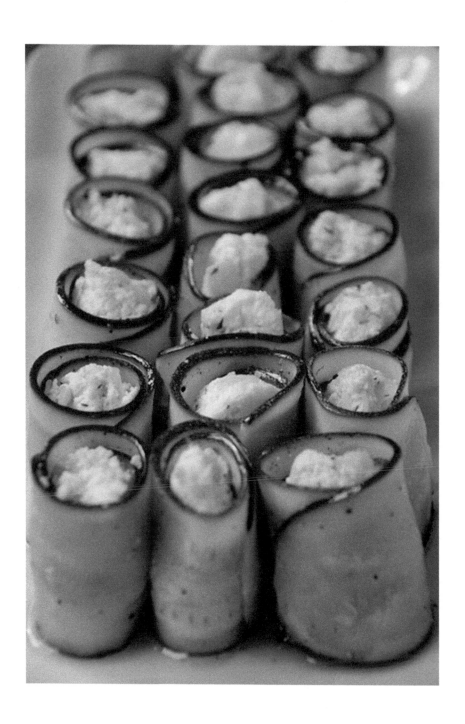

Lemon Salmon Bites

Servings: 4

Cooking Time: 2 Hours

Ingredients:

- 4 salmon fillets, skinless, boneless and cubed
- 1 lemon, sliced
- 1 cup low-sodium veggie stock
- 2 tablespoons chili pepper
- Juice of 1 lemon
- 1 teaspoon basil, dried
- 1 teaspoon sweet paprika
- Salt and black pepper to the taste

Directions:

1. In your slow cooker, mix chili pepper with lemon juice, stock, paprika, basil, pepper and salmon, cover and cook on High for 2 hours.
2. Divide salmon into bowls drizzle sauce from the pot all over and serve.

Nutrition Info:

Calories 284, Fat 12.8g, Cholesterol 78mg, Sodium 380mg, Carbohydrate 7g, Fiber 1.1g, Sugars 3.4g, Protein 35.7g, Potassium 753mg

American Fondue

Servings: 12 Servings

Ingredients:

- 1 can (10.5 ounces, or 295 g) Cheddar cheese soup
- 2 cups (225 g) shredded Cheddar cheese
- 2 cups (220 g) shredded Swiss cheese
- 12 ounces (355 ml) beer or 1½ cups (355 ml) apple cider
- ½ teaspoon hot pepper sauce
- 2 drops liquid smoke

Directions:

1. Place all ingredients in slow cooker. Stir to mix. Cover and cook on low for 2 hours. After 1 hour of cooking time, stir. Before serving, whisk to blend. Serve with bread sticks or vegetables for dipping.

Nutrition Info:

Per serving: 63 g water; 215 calories (67% from fat, 25% from protein, 8% from carb); 13 g protein; 15 g total fat; 10 g saturated fat; 4 g monounsaturated fat; 0 g polyunsaturated fat; 4 g carb; 0 g fiber; 1 g sugar; 277 mg phosphorus; 400 mg calcium; 0 mg iron; 336 mg sodium; 85 mg potassium; 481 IU vitamin A; 121 mg ATE vitamin E; 0 mg vitamin C; 49 mg cholesterol

Cream Cheese and Kale Dip

Servings: 4

Cooking Time: 1 Hour

Ingredients:

- 1 pound baby kale
- 1 cup coconut cream
- 2 spring onions, chopped
- 1 cup low-fat cream cheese
- 1 scallion, chopped
- 2 tablespoons mint leaves, chopped
- A pinch of cayenne pepper
- A pinch of red pepper flakes, crushed

Directions:

1. In your slow cooker, combine the kale with the cream, spring onions and the other ingredients, put the lid on and cook on Low for 1 hour.
2. Blend using an immersion blender, divide into bowls and serve as a party dip.

Nutrition Info:

Calories 404, Fat 35.2g, Cholesterol 64mg, Sodium 229mg, Carbohydrate 17.4g, Fiber 4.4g, Sugars 2.3g, Protein 10g, Potassium 262mg

Butterscotch Dip

Servings: 16 Servings

Ingredients:

- 20 ounces (560 g) butterscotch chips
- 5 ounces (150 ml) fat-free evaporated milk
- 1 tablespoon (15 ml) rum extract

Directions:

1. Combine all ingredients in slow cooker and cook on low until chips are soft, about 1 hour. Stir.

Nutrition Info:

Per serving: 9 g water; 145 calories (7% from fat, 2% from protein, 91% from carb); 1 g protein; 1 g total fat; 1 g saturated fat; 0 g monounsaturated fat; 0 g polyunsaturated fat; 33 g carb; 0 g fiber; 30 g sugar; 18 mg phosphorus; 27 mg calcium; 0 mg iron; 149 mg sodium; 30 mg potassium; 70 IU vitamin A; 20 mg ATE vitamin E; 0 mg vitamin C; 4 mg cholesterol

Beer Barbecued Meatballs

Servings: 36 Servings

Ingredients:

- 3 pounds (1.4 kg) lean ground beef
- 1 cup (160 g) chopped onion, divided
- ½ cup (60 g) dry bread crumbs
- ¾ cup (175 ml) egg substitute
- 12 ounces (355 ml) beer
- 6 ounces (175 ml) spicy vegetable juice, such as V-8
- 1 teaspoon lemon juice
- 1 teaspoon hot pepper sauce
- 14 ounces (390 g) no-salt-added ketchup
- 1 teaspoon horseradish
- 1 teaspoon Worcestershire sauce

Directions:

1. Combine ground beef, ½ cup (80 g) onions, bread crumbs, and egg substitute. Make the mixture into small meatballs. Cook meatballs in a large skillet, turning to brown all sides, or bake in a 375°F (190°C, or gas mark 5) oven until browned, about 30 minutes. Drain meatballs and discard fat. In a saucepan, combine remaining ingredients. Simmer

31

for 15 minutes. Put meatballs and sauce into slow cooker. Cover and cook on low for 3 to 6 hours. Makes about 6 dozen meatballs.

Nutrition Info:

Per serving: 53 g water; 116 calories (54% from fat, 29% from protein, 17% from carb); 8 g protein; 7 g total fat; 3 g saturated fat; 3 g monounsaturated fat; 0 g polyunsaturated fat; 5 g carb; 0 g fiber; 3 g sugar; 69 mg phosphorus; 12 mg calcium; 1 mg iron; 42 mg sodium; 190 mg potassium; 198 IU vitamin A; 0 mg ATE vitamin E; 4 mg vitamin C; 26 mg cholesterol

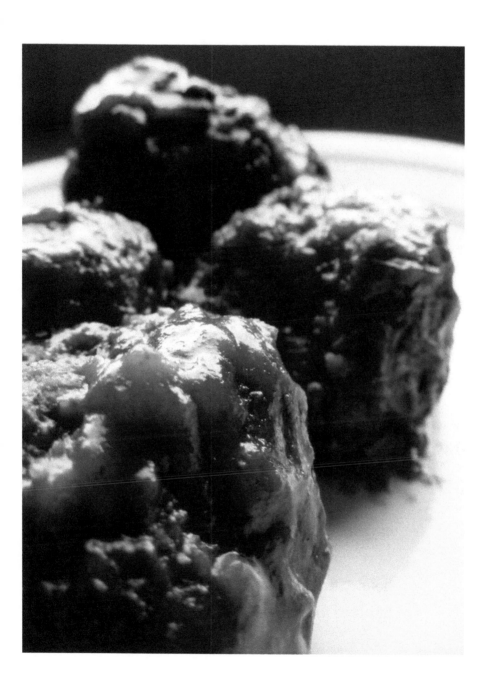

Sweet And Spicy Nuts

Servings: 22 Servings

Ingredients:

- 1 cup (140 g) unsalted cashews
- 1 cup (145 g) unsalted almonds, toasted
- 1 cup (100 g) unsalted pecan halves, toasted
- ½ cup (100 g) sugar
- 1/3 cup (75 g) unsalted butter, melted
- 1 teaspoon ground ginger
- ½ teaspoon cinnamon
- ¼ teaspoon cloves
- ¼ teaspoon cayenne pepper

Directions:

1. Place nuts in a slow cooker. In a small bowl, combine sugar, butter, ginger, cinnamon, cloves, and cayenne pepper. Add to cooker, stirring to coat nuts. Cover and cook on low for 2 hours, stirring after 1 hour. Stir nuts again. Spread in a single layer on buttered foil; let cool for at least 1 hour.

Nutrition Info:

Per serving: 1 g water; 189 calories (75% from fat, 7% from protein, 19% from carb); 3 g protein; 17 g total fat; 3 g saturated fat; 9 g monounsaturated fat; 4 g polyunsaturated fat; 9 g carb; 2 g fiber; 6 g sugar; 92 mg phosphorus; 29 mg calcium; 1 mg iron; 2 mg sodium; 129 mg potassium; 109 IU vitamin A; 23 mg ATE vitamin E; 0 mg vitamin C; 7 mg cholesterol

Sour Cream Dip

Servings: 4

Cooking Time: 2 Hours

Ingredients:

- 1 bunch spinach leaves, roughly chopped
- ¾ cup low-fat sour cream
- 1 scallion, sliced
- 2 tablespoons mint leaves, chopped
- Black pepper to the taste

Directions:

1. In your slow cooker, mix the spinach with the scallion, mint, cream and black pepper, cover, cook on High for 2 hours, stir well, divide into bowls and serve.

Nutrition Info:

Calories 121, Fat 9.7g, Cholesterol 19mg, Sodium 147mg, Carbohydrate 6.3g, Fiber 2.2g, Sugars 1g, Protein 4g, Potassium 560mg

Hot Crab Dip

Servings: 16 Servings

Ingredients:

- 16 ounces (455 g) fat-free cream cheese
- 4 ounces (115 g) pepper jack cheese, shredded
- 2 teaspoons Worcestershire sauce
- 1½ cups (150 g) scallions, chopped
- ¼ cup (15 g) fresh parsley, chopped
- 1 pound (455 g) crab meat
- ½ cup (120 ml) skim milk

Directions:

1. Cook together in slow cooker on low heat until dip reaches desired consistency, about 2 hours.

Nutrition Info:

Per serving: 60 g water; 123 calories (55% from fat, 34% from protein, 11% from carb); 10 g protein; 7 g total fat; 5 g saturated fat; 2 g monounsaturated fat; 0 g polyunsaturated fat; 3 g carb; 0 g fiber; 1 g sugar; 150 mg phosphorus; 127 mg calcium; 1 mg iron; 216 mg sodium; 194 mg potassium; 437 IU vitamin A; 70 mg ATE vitamin E; 5 mg vitamin C; 44 mg cholesterol

Herbed Zucchini Salad

Servings: 4

Cooking Time: 1 Hour

Ingredients:

- 2 pounds shrimp, peeled and deveined
- ½ cup coconut cream
- 2 tablespoons lime juice
- 1 tablespoon avocado oil
- ½ pound zucchinis, cubed
- 1 cup cherry tomatoes, halved
- 2 tablespoons chives, chopped
- ½ teaspoon oregano, chopped
- 2 garlic cloves, minced

Directions:

1. In the slow cooker, combine the shrimp with the zucchinis, cream and the other ingredients, put the lid on and cook on High for 1 hour.
2. Divide into bowls and serve as an appetizer.

Nutrition Info:

Calories 365, Fat 11.7g, Cholesterol 478mg, Sodium 566mg, Carbohydrate 10.3g, Fiber 2.2g, Sugars 3.4g, Protein 53.7g, Potassium 752mg

Asian Chicken Wings

Servings: 16 Servings

Ingredients:

- 3 pounds (1.4 kg) chicken wings
- 1 cup (160 g) chopped onion
- 1 cup (235 ml) low sodium soy sauce
- 1 cup (225 g) brown sugar
- 2 teaspoons ground ginger
- ½ teaspoon minced garlic
- ¼ cup (60 ml) sherry

Directions:

1. Rinse chicken wings; pat dry. Cut off and discard wing tips and then cut each wing at the joint to make two sections. Place wings on a lightly oiled broiler pan. Broil about 4 inches from the heat for 10 minutes on each side or until chicken wings are nicely browned. Transfer chicken wings to slow cooker. In a bowl, combine chopped onion, soy sauce, brown sugar, ginger, garlic, and sherry. Pour sauce over chicken wings. Cover and cook on low for 4 to 5 hours or on high for 2 to 2½ hours. Stir wings once about halfway through cooking. Serve directly from slow

cooker, keeping temperature on low. Makes about 32 wing pieces.

Nutrition Info:

Per serving: 87 g water; 178 calories (16% from fat, 46% from protein, 38% from carb); 20 g protein; 3 g total fat; 1 g saturated fat; 1 g monounsaturated fat; 1 g polyunsaturated fat; 16 g carb; 0 g fiber; 14 g sugar; 156 mg phosphorus; 28 mg calcium; 1 mg iron; 125 mg sodium; 263 mg potassium; 51 IU vitamin A; 15 mg ATE vitamin E; 2 mg vitamin C; 48 mg cholesterol

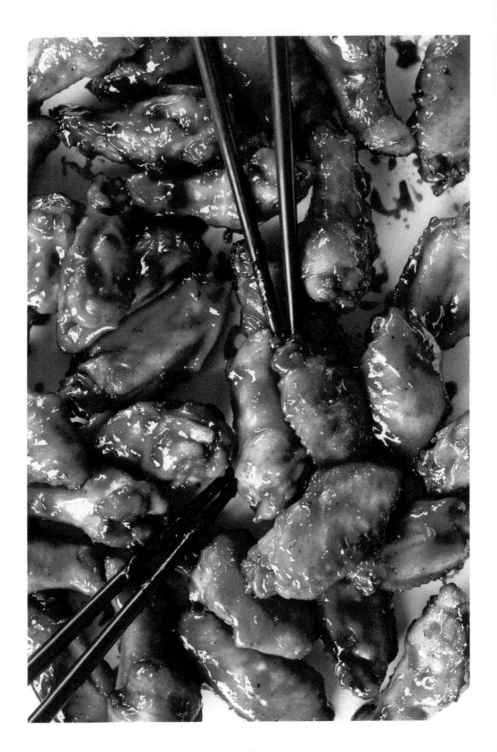

Cranberries Salad

Servings: 12

Cooking Time: 6 Hours

Ingredients:

- 2 cups sweet onions, sliced
- 1 apple, peeled, cored and cut into wedges
- ½ cup cranberries
- ¼ cup balsamic vinegar
- 2 tablespoons olive oil
- 1 tablespoon stevia
- ½ teaspoon orange zest, grated
- 7 ounces low-fat cheddar cheese, shredded

Directions:

1. In your slow cooker, mix apples with cranberries, onions, oil, vinegar, stevia and orange zest, stir, cover and cook on Low for 6 hours.
2. Divide into bowls, sprinkle the cheese on top and serve.

Nutrition Info:

Calories 108, Fat 7.9g, Cholesterol 17mg, Sodium 104mg, Carbohydrate 5.7g, Fiber 1g, Sugars .3g, Protein 4.4g, Potassium 76mg

Cherry Tomatoes and Spinach Salsa

Servings: 4

Cooking Time: 4 Hours

Ingredients:

- 2 cups canned black beans, no-salt added, drained and rinsed
- 1 cup corn
- 1 cup kalamata olives, pitted and halved
- 1 cup baby spinach
- 1 cup cherry tomatoes, halved
- 1 cup spring onions, chopped
- 1 cup low-sodium veggie stock
- 1 tablespoon balsamic vinegar
- 1 tablespoon avocado oil
- 2 tablespoons lemon juice

Directions:

1. In the slow cooker, combine the black beans with the corn, olives and the other ingredients except the

spinach, put the lid on and cook on Low for 3 hours and 30 minutes.

2. Add the spinach, cook the mix for 30 minutes more on Low, divide into bowls and serve as an appetizer.

Nutrition Info:

Calories 431, Fat 6.1g, Cholesterol 0mg, Sodium 353mg, Carbohydrate 76.4g, Fiber 18.4g, Sugars 5.5g, Protein 23.7g, Potassium 1786mg

Salmon Appetizer Mix

Servings: 4

Cooking Time: 9 Hours

Ingredients:

- 16 ounces baby carrots
- 4 salmon fillets, boneless and cubed
- 3 tablespoons olive oil
- ¼ cup low-sodium veggie stock
- ½ teaspoon dill, chopped
- 4 garlic cloves, minced
- A pinch of black pepper

Directions:

1. In your slow cooker, mix oil with carrots, stock and garlic, stir, cover and cook on Low for 7 hours.
2. Add salmon, pepper and dill, cover, cook on Low for 2 hours more, divide everything into bowls and serve as an appetizer

Nutrition Info:

Calories 371, Fat 21.7g, Cholesterol 78mg, Sodium 176mg, Carbohydrate 10.5g, Fiber 3.4g, Sugars 5.5g, Protein 35.5g, Potassium 969mg

Beet And Basil Spread

Servings: 8

Cooking Time: 4 Hours

Ingredients:

- 6 beets, peeled and chopped
- 1 yellow onion, chopped
- 1 cup low-sodium veggie stock
- ¼ cup lemon juice
- 2 tablespoons olive oil
- 7 celery ribs
- 8 garlic cloves, minced
- 1 bunch basil, chopped
- Black pepper to the taste

Directions:

1. Grease your slow cooker with the oil, add celery, onion, beets, garlic, stock, lemon juice, basil and pepper, stir, cover and cook on Low for 4 hours.
2. Blend using an immersion blender, divide into bowls and serve.

Nutrition Info:

Calories 171, Fat 7.9g, Cholesterol 0mg, Sodium 250mg, Carbohydrate 23g, Fiber 5g, Sugars 14.9g, Protein 4.4g, Potassium 727mg

Mexican Dip

Servings: 20 Servings

Ingredients:

- 1 pound (455 g) extra-lean ground beef
- 1 cup (160 g) chopped onion
- 2 cups (476 g) refried beans
- 1 tablespoon (7 g) Salt-Free Mexican Seasoning
- 1 cup (230 g) fat-free sour cream
- ½ cup (58 g) shredded Cheddar cheese

Directions:

1. Brown beef and onions in a skillet over medium-high heat and stir in refried beans and Mexican seasoning. Place in bottom of slow cooker. Spread sour cream over and sprinkle with cheese. Cover and cook on low for 1½ to 2 hours.

Nutrition Info:

Per serving: 52 g water; 110 calories (56% from fat, 25% from protein, 19% from carb); 7 g protein; 7 g total fat; 3 g saturated fat; 3 g monounsaturated fat; 0 g polyunsaturated fat; 5 g carb; 1 g fiber; 0 g sugar; 84 mg phosphorus; 49 mg calcium; 1 mg iron;

46 mg sodium; 162 mg potassium; 78 IU vitamin A; 21 mg ATE vitamin E; 2 mg vitamin C; 26 mg cholesterol

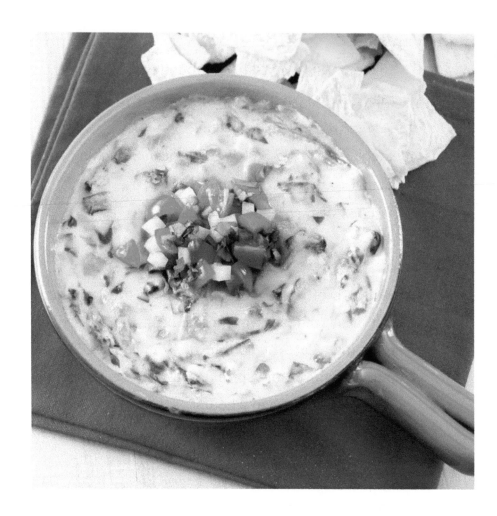

Creamy Spinach Dip

Servings: 4

Cooking Time: 1 Hour

Ingredients:
- 10 ounces spinach leaves
- 8 ounces water chestnuts, chopped
- 1 cup coconut cream
- 1 garlic clove, minced
- Black pepper to the taste

Directions:
1. In your slow cooker, mix coconut cream with spinach, chestnuts, black pepper and garlic, stir, cover, cook on High for 1 hour, blend with an immersion blender, divide into bowls and serve as a dip

Nutrition Info:

Calories 248, Fat 15.1g, Cholesterol 0mg, Sodium 115mg, Carbohydrate 26.6g, Fiber 2.9g, Sugars 2.7g, Protein 4.8g, Potassium 743mg

Creamy Mexican Beef And Bean Dip

Servings: 32 Servings

Ingredients:

- 1 pound (455 g) lean ground beef
- ½ cup (80 g) chopped onion
- ¾ cup (175 g) mild picante sauce
- 2 cups (512 g) cooked kidney beans
- 1 cup (230 g) sour cream
- ½ teaspoon chili powder
- 8 ounces (225 g) Cheddar cheese, shredded
- Jalapeños or mild chili peppers, chopped, to taste

Directions:

1. Cook ground beef with onion in a skillet over medium-high heat; drain. Mix beef mixture and remaining ingredients together in slow cooker and cook on low about 3 to 4 hours. Serve with your favorite vegetables or chips.

Nutrition Info:

Per serving: 32 g water; 88 calories (59% from fat, 26% from protein, 15% from carb); 6 g protein; 6 g total fat; 3 g saturated fat; 2 g monounsaturated fat; 0 g polyunsaturated fat; 3 g carb; 1 g fiber; 0 g sugar; 80 mg phosphorus; 66 mg calcium; 1 mg iron; 78 mg sodium; 103 mg potassium; 133 IU vitamin A; 26 mg ATE vitamin E; 1 mg vitamin C; 20 mg cholesterol

Basil Pecans

Servings: 5

Cooking Time: 2 Hours

Ingredients:

- 1 pound pecans, halved
- 1 tablespoon chili powder
- 2 tablespoons olive oil
- 1 teaspoon basil, dried
- 1 teaspoon oregano, dried
- ½ teaspoon onion powder
- ¼ teaspoon garlic powder
- 1 teaspoon rosemary, dried

Directions:

1. In your slow cooker, mix pecans with oil, basil, chili powder, oregano, garlic powder, onion powder and rosemary, toss, cover and cook on Low for 2 hours.
2. Divide into bowls and serve as a snack.

Nutrition Info:

Calories 688, Fat 70.7g, Cholesterol 0mg, Sodium 16mg, Carbohydrate 14.4g, Fiber 10.5g, Sugars 3.5g, Protein 10g, Potassium 416mg

Dill Meat Rolls

Servings: 4

Cooking Time: 8 Hours

Ingredients:

- 25 ounces tomato sauce, no-salt-added
- 1 cup cauliflower rice
- 1 green cabbage head, leaves separated
- ½ cup onion, chopped
- 2 ounces white mushrooms, chopped
- ½ pounds beef meat, minced
- 2 garlic cloves, minced
- ¼ cup water
- 2 tablespoons dill, chopped
- 1 tablespoon olive oil
- A pinch of black pepper

Directions:

1. In a bowl, mix beef with onion, cauliflower, mushrooms, garlic, dill and pepper and stir.
2. Arrange cabbage leaves on a working surface, divide the beef mix and wrap them well.

3. Add sauce and water to your slow cooker, stir, add cabbage rolls, cover, cook on Low for 8 hours, arrange the rolls on a platter and serve them as an appetizer.

Nutrition Info:

Calories 243, Fat 8.3g, Cholesterol 43mg, Sodium 1033mg, Carbohydrate 24.8g, Fiber 7.8g, Sugars 15.1g, Protein 21.5g, Potassium 1211mg

Sriracha Dip

Servings: 10

Cooking Time: 3 Hours And 30 Minutes

Ingredients:

- 8 ounces coconut cream
- 1 pound chicken breast, skinless, boneless and sliced
- ¼ cup low-sodium chicken stock
- 3 tablespoons jalapeno pepper powder
- 2 tablespoons stevia
- 1 teaspoon chili powder

Directions:

1. In your slow cooker, mix chicken with jalapeno pepper, stock, stevia and chili powder, stir, cover and cook on High for 3 hours.
2. Shred meat, return to pot, add coconut cream, cover, cook on High for 30 minutes more, divide into bowls and serve.

Nutrition Info:

Calories 105, Fat 6.6g, Cholesterol 29mg, Sodium 33mg, Carbohydrate 3.5g, Fiber 0.6g, Sugars 0.8g, Protein 10.2g, Potassium 232mg

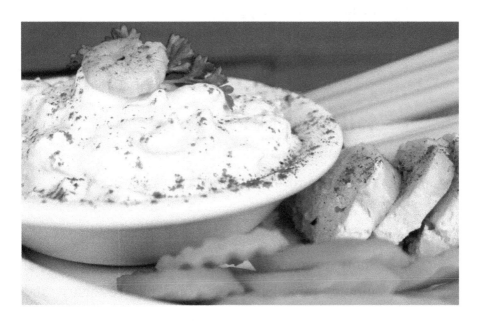

Walnuts And Seeds Bowl

Servings: 1 0

Cooking Time: 3 Hours

Ingredients:

- 1 cup walnuts, chopped
- 1 cup pumpkin seeds
- Cooking spray
- 2 tablespoons olive oil
- 2 tablespoons dill, dried
- 1 tablespoon lemon peel, grated
- 1 teaspoon rosemary, dried

Directions:

1. Spray your slow cooker with cooking spray, add walnuts, pumpkin seeds, oil, dill, rosemary and lemon peel, toss, cover, cook on Low for 3 hours, divide into bowls and serve as a snack.

Nutrition Info:

Calories 179, Fat 16.6g, Cholesterol 0mg, Sodium 4mg, Carbohydrate 4.3g, Fiber 1.6g, Sugars 0.3g, Protein 6.5g, Potassium 200mg

Hot Cheesy Crabmeat Dip

Servings: 8 Servings

Ingredients:

- 10 ounces (280 g) sharp Cheddar cheese
- 8 ounces (225 g) fat-free cream cheese
- ½ cup (120 ml) skim milk
- ½ cup (120 ml) dry white wine
- 8 ounces (225 g) crabmeat

Directions:

1. Spray the bottom and sides of slow cooker with nonstick cooking spray. Place the two cheeses and milk in prepared slow cooker. Cook 1 to 2 hours. Add wine and crabmeat and stir to combine; cover and cook for 1 hour longer.

Nutrition Info:

Per serving: 79 g water; 255 calories (64% from fat, 30% from protein, 6% from carb); 18 g protein; 17 g total fat; 11 g saturated fat; 5 g monounsaturated fat; 1 g polyunsaturated fat; 4 g carb; 0 g fiber; 0 g sugar; 316 mg phosphorus; 339 mg calcium; 1 mg iron; 408 mg sodium; 227 mg potassium; 581 IU vitamin A; 153 mg ATE vitamin E; 1 mg vitamin C; 79 mg cholesterol

Sweet And Spicy Bratwurst

Servings: 16 Servings

Ingredients:

- 2 pounds (910 g) bratwurst, cut in 1-inch (2.5 cm) pieces
- 2 tablespoons (28 ml) oil
- 1 cup (160 g) chopped onions
- ¼ cup (60 g) brown sugar
- 4 teaspoons (11 g) cornstarch
- ¼ cup (60 ml) cider vinegar
- ¼ cup (44 g) mustard
- 4 teaspoons (20 g) horseradish

Directions:

1. In a skillet over medium heat, brown meat in oil and remove, sautéing onions in remaining oil. Drain oil. Transfer to slow cooker. Combine remaining ingredients and add to cooker. Cook on low for 3 hours.

Nutrition Info:

Per serving: 51 g water; 145 calories (60% from fat, 24% from protein, 17% from carb); 9 g protein; 10 g total fat; 0 g saturated fat; 5 g monounsaturated fat; 1 g polyunsaturated fat; 6 g carb; 0 g fiber; 5 g sugar; 79 mg phosphorus; 17 mg calcium; 1 mg iron; 563 mg sodium; 179 mg potassium; 4 IU vitamin A; 0 mg ATE vitamin E; 1 mg vitamin C; 32 mg cholesterol

Sweet And Sour Chicken Wings

Servings: 16 Servings

Ingredients:

- 3 pounds (1.4 kg) chicken wings
- ¼ cup (60 ml) balsamic vinegar
- 1 cup (330 g) apricot preserves
- 1 cup (240 g) no-salt-added ketchup
- 3 tablespoons (45 g) horseradish
- 1 cup (160 g) finely chopped onion
- 1 teaspoon hot pepper sauce, or to taste

Directions:

1. Pat the chicken wings dry and place them in the slow cooker. In a bowl, mix together remaining ingredients. Taste and adjust seasonings. Pour the sauce over the wings. Cover the slow cooker and cook on low until the chicken is tender, about 4 to 5 hours.

Nutrition Info:

Per serving: 95 g water; 183 calories (16% from fat, 43% from protein, 42% from carb); 19 g protein; 3 g total fat; 1 g saturated fat; 1 g monounsaturated fat; 1 g polyunsaturated fat; 19 g carb;

1 g fiber; 14 g sugar; 145 mg phosphorus; 22 mg calcium; 1 mg iron; 90 mg sodium; 262 mg potassium; 195 IU vitamin A; 15 mg ATE vitamin E; 6 mg vitamin C; 48 mg cholesterol

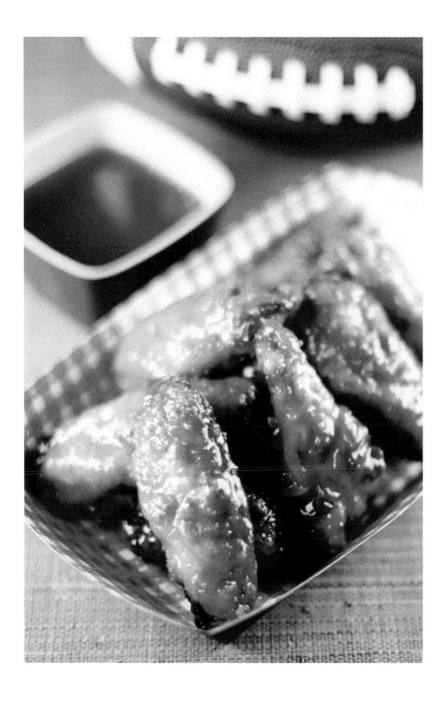

Garlic and Tomato Appetizer

Servings: 4

Cooking Time: 2 Hours

Ingredients:

- 2 teaspoons olive oil
- 8 tomatoes, chopped
- 1 garlic clove, minced
- ¼ cup basil, chopped
- 4 Italian whole wheat bread slices, toasted
- 3 tablespoons low-sodium veggie stock
- Black pepper to the taste

Directions:

1. In your slow cooker, mix tomatoes with basil, garlic, oil, stock and black pepper, stir, cover, cook on High for 2 hours and then leave aside to cool down.
2. Divide this mix on the toasted bread and serve as an appetizer.

Nutrition Info:

Calories 158, Fat 4.1g, Cholesterol 0mg, Sodium 251mg, Carbohydrate 26.3g, Fiber 4.5g, Sugars 6.9g, Protein 5.9g, Potassium 590mg

Oregano Salsa

Servings: 4

Cooking Time: 7 Hours

Ingredients:

- 3 cups eggplant, cubed
- 4 garlic cloves, minced
- 6 ounces green olives, pitted and sliced
- 1 and ½ cups tomatoes, chopped
- 2 teaspoons balsamic vinegar
- 1 tablespoon oregano, chopped
- Black pepper to the taste

Directions:

1. In your slow cooker, mix tomatoes with eggplant, green olives, garlic, vinegar, oregano and pepper, toss, cover, cook on Low for 7 hours, divide into small bowls and serve as an appetizer.

Nutrition Info:

Calories 78, Fat 3.6g, Cholesterol 0mg, Sodium 443mg, Carbohydrate 11.2g, Fiber 4.6g, Sugars 4.2g, Protein 2g, Potassium 337mg

Cocktail Meatballs

Servings: 12 Servings

Ingredients:

- 1 pound (455 g) lean ground beef
- ½ cup (60 g) bread crumbs
- 1/3 cup (55 g) minced onion
- ¼ cup (60 ml) skim milk
- ¼ cup (60 ml) egg substitute
- 1 tablespoon (4 g) fresh parsley, chopped
- 1/8 teaspoon black pepper
- ½ teaspoon Worcestershire sauce
- 2 tablespoons (28 ml) olive oil
- 1 cup (275 g) chili sauce
- ½ cup (170 g) grape jelly

Directions:

1. Mix the first 8 ingredients (through Worcestershire sauce) and make into bite-size meatballs. Heat the oil in a skillet and brown meatballs in the oil. Transfer to the slow cooker. Mix the chili sauce and the jelly in a saucepan over low heat until melted. Add to meatballs and stir until coated. Cook on low for 4 to 6 hours.

Nutrition Info:

Per serving: 60 g water; 181 calories (47% from fat, 20% from protein, 33% from carb); 9 g protein; 9 g total fat; 3 g saturated fat; 5 g monounsaturated fat; 1 g polyunsaturated fat; 15 g carb; 1 g fiber; 8 g sugar; 77 mg phosphorus; 30 mg calcium; 1 mg iron; 60 mg sodium; 163 mg potassium; 390 IU vitamin A; 3 mg ATE vitamin E; 6 mg vitamin C; 26 mg cholesterol

Cream Cheese Dip

Servings: 4

Cooking Time: 2 Hours

Ingredients:

- 1 pound zucchinis, grated
- ½ cup coconut cream
- 1 teaspoon turmeric powder
- 8 ounces fat-free cream cheese
- 2 tablespoons chives, chopped
- 1 tablespoon dill, chopped

Directions:

1. In your slow cooker, combine the zucchinis with the cream, turmeric and the other ingredients, put the lid on and cook on Low for 2 hours.
2. Divide into bowls and serve as a party dip.

Nutrition Info:

Calories 289, Fat 27.2g, Cholesterol 62mg, Sodium 186mg, Carbohydrate 7.8g, Fiber 2.2g, Sugars 3.1g, Protein 6.6g, Potassium 488mg

Honey Chicken Wings

Servings: 16 Servings

Ingredients:

- 3 pounds (1.4 kg) chicken wings
- 1 cup (340 g) honey
- ½ cup (120 ml) low sodium soy sauce
- 2 tablespoons (28 ml) olive oil
- 2 tablespoons (30 g) no-salt-added ketchup
- ½ teaspoon minced garlic

Directions:

1. Cut off and discard chicken wing tips. Cut each wing into 2 parts. Combine remaining ingredients and mix well. Place wings in slow cooker and pour sauce over. Cook 6 to 7 hours on low.

Nutrition Info:

Per serving: 74 g water; 193 calories (22% from fat, 40% from protein, 38% from carb); 19 g protein; 5 g total fat; 1 g saturated fat; 2 g monounsaturated fat; 1 g polyunsaturated fat; 19 g carb; 0 g fiber; 18 g sugar; 142 mg phosphorus; 14 mg calcium; 1 mg iron; 95 mg sodium; 198 mg potassium; 68 IU vitamin A; 15 mg ATE vitamin E; 1 mg vitamin C; 48 mg cholesterol

Salmon And Cherry Tomatoes Salad

Servings: 4

Cooking Time: 2 Hour s

Ingredients:

- 1 pound salmon fillets, boneless and roughly cubed
- Juice of 1 orange
- 1 mango, peeled and cubed
- 1 cup baby spinach
- 1 cup cherry tomatoes, halved
- 1 teaspoon coriander, ground
- 2 tablespoons olive oil
- 2 spring onions, chopped
- 1 red onion, sliced
- 1 Serrano chili pepper, chopped
- ¼ cup cilantro, chopped

Directions:

1. In the slow cooker, combine the salmon with the orange juice, mango and the other ingredients, put the lid on and cook on Low for 2 hours.

2. Divide between appetizer plates and serve.

Nutrition Info:

Calories 300, Fat 14.5g, Cholesterol 50mg, Sodium 61mg, Carbohydrate 20g, Fiber 2.9g, Sugars 15.8g, Protein 23.9g, Potassium 829mg

Nutmeg Endive Salad

Servings: 4

Cooking Time: 3 Hours

Ingredients:

- 1 cup low-sodium chicken stock
- 4 endives, trimmed
- 14 ounces coconut cream
- 4 slices low-sodium ham, chopped
- 2 tablespoons olive oil
- ½ teaspoon nutmeg, ground
- Black pepper to the taste

Directions:

1. In your slow cooker, mix endives with stock, pepper, oil, ham, nutmeg and coconut cream, cover and cook on High for 3 hours.
2. Divide into small bowls and serve as an appetizer.

Nutrition Info:

Calories 347, Fat 33.5g, Cholesterol 16mg, Sodium 475mg, Carbohydrate 8.4g, Fiber 3.4g, Sugars .3.9g, Protein 7.6g, Potassium 421mg

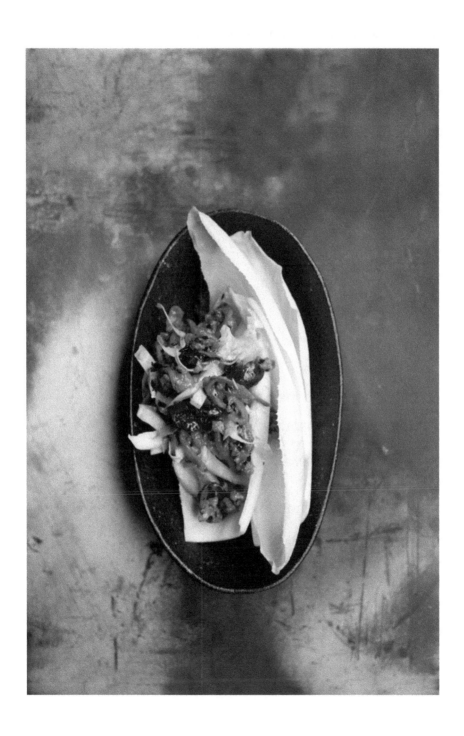

Salmon And Shallot Salad

Servings: 4

Cooking Time: 1 Hour

Ingredients:

- 4 medium salmon fillets, boneless and cubed
- 2 shallots, chopped
- 1 cup low sodium veggie stock
- 1 lettuce head, torn
- ¼ cup olive oil+ 1 tablespoon
- 2 tablespoons lemon juice
- 3 tablespoons parsley, finely chopped
- Black pepper to the taste

Directions:

1. Brush salmon fillets with 1 tablespoon of oil, season with pepper, put them in your slow cooker, add stock, cover and cook on High for 1 hour.
2. Transfer salmon to a salad bowl, add shallots, lemon juice, lettuce, the rest of the oil and parsley, toss and serve as an appetizer.

Nutrition Info:

Calories 407, Fat 28.3g, Cholesterol 78mg, Sodium 178mg, Carbohydrate 5g, Fiber 0.7g, Sugars 1.7g, Protein 35.2g, Potassium 840mg

Peppercorns Asparagus

Servings: 6

Cooking Time: 2 Hours

Ingredients:

- 3 cups asparagus spears, halved
- 3 garlic cloves, sliced
- 1 tablespoon dill
- ¼ cup white wine vinegar
- ¼ cup apple cider vinegar
- 2 cloves
- 1 cup water
- ¼ teaspoon red pepper flakes
- 8 black peppercorns
- 1 teaspoon coriander seeds

Directions:

1. In your slow cooker, mix the asparagus with the cider vinegar, white vinegar, dill, cloves, water, garlic, pepper flakes, peppercorns and coriander, cover and cook on High for 2 hours.
2. Drain asparagus, transfer it to bowls and serve as a snack.

Nutrition Info:

Calories 20, Fat 0.1g, Cholesterol 0mg, Sodium 4mg, Carbohydrate 3.6g, Fiber 1.6g, Sugars 1.3g, Protein 1.7g, Potassium 170mg

Broccoli Dip

Servings: 20 Servings

Ingredients:

- 10 ounces (280 g) frozen broccoli, chopped
- ½ cup (50 g) chopped celery
- 1 cup (160 g) chopped onion
- 2 tablespoons (28 g) unsalted butter
- 4 ounces (115 g) mushroom, sliced
- 8 ounces (225 g) fat-free cream cheese
- 10 ounces (280 g) low-sodium cream of mushroom soup
- 6 ounces (170 g) water chestnuts, sliced
- 2 teaspoons Worcestershire sauce

Directions:

1. Cook broccoli until tender. In a skillet over medium-high heat, sauté celery and onion in butter until tender. Place broccoli and sautéed vegetables in slow cooker; add mushrooms, cream cheese, and cream of mushroom soup. Stir well and heat on low until cheese is melted. Add water chestnuts and Worcestershire sauce. Serve warm in the slow cooker.

Nutrition Info:

Per serving: 54 g water; 62 calories (49% from fat, 14% from protein, 38% from carb); 2 g protein; 3 g total fat; 2 g saturated fat; 1 g monounsaturated fat; 0 g polyunsaturated fat; 6 g carb; 1 g fiber; 1 g sugar; 47 mg phosphorus; 26 mg calcium; 0 mg iron; 101 mg sodium; 207 mg potassium; 214 IU vitamin A; 30 mg ATE vitamin E; 15 mg vitamin C; 10 mg cholesterol

Creole Shrimps

Servings: 4

Cooking Time: 1 Hour

Ingredients:

- 1 pound jumbo shrimp, peeled and deveined
- 1 and ½ cups low-sodium chicken stock
- Juice of 1 lemon
- 2 teaspoons Creole seasoning
- 4 teaspoons cider vinegar
- 4 teaspoons avocado oil
- Black pepper to the taste

Directions:

1. Grease your slow cooker with the oil, add shrimp, vinegar, stock, lemon juice, pepper and Creole seasoning, cover, cook on High for 1 hour, transfer the shrimp to a platter and serve as an appetizer.

Nutrition Info:

Calories 98, Fat 0.9g, Cholesterol 233mg, Sodium 1952mg, Carbohydrate 1.2g, Fiber 0.3g, Sugars 2.7g, Protein 20.8g, Potassium 33mg

Parmesan Stuffed Mushrooms

Servings: 20

Cooking Time: 5 Hours

Ingredients:

- 20 mushrooms, stems removed
- 2 cups basil, chopped
- 1 cup tomato sauce, no-salt-added
- 2 tablespoons parsley, chopped
- ¼ cup low-fat parmesan, grated
- 1 and ½ cups whole wheat breadcrumbs
- 1 tablespoon garlic, minced
- ¼ cup low-fat butter, melted
- 2 teaspoons lemon juice
- 1 tablespoon olive oil

Directions:

1. In a bowl, mix butter with breadcrumbs and parsley, stir well and leave aside.
2. In your blender, mix basil with oil, parmesan, garlic and lemon juice and pulse really well.

3. Stuff mushrooms with this mix, pour the tomato sauce on top, sprinkle breadcrumbs mix at the end, cover and cook on Low for 5 hours.

4. Arrange mushrooms on a platter and serve.

Nutrition Info:

Calories 51, Fat 1.1g, Cholesterol 0mg, Sodium 109mg, Carbohydrate 9g, Fiber 1.2g, Sugars 1.1g, Protein 2.2g, Potassium 109mg

Cinnamon Nuts Mix

Servings: 20

Cooking Time: 4 Hours

Ingredients:

- 4 tablespoons olive oil
- 1-ounce Italian seasoning
- Cayenne pepper to the taste
- 2 cups almonds
- 2 cups walnuts
- 2 cups cashews
- 1 teaspoon cinnamon powder

Directions:

1. In your slow cooker, mix oil with Italian seasoning, cinnamon, cayenne, cashews, almonds and walnuts, toss well, cover, cook on Low for 4 hours, divide into bowls and serve as a snack.

Nutrition Info:

Calories 240, Fat 21.7g, Cholesterol 1mg, Sodium 3mg, Carbohydrate 8.1g, Fiber 2.5g, Sugars 1.4g, Protein 7.2g, Potassium 213mg

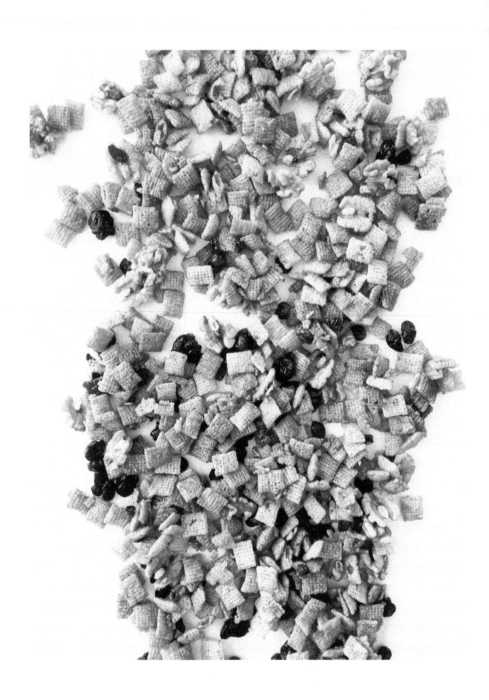

Almond Flour Sticks

Servings: 4

Cooking Time: 2 Hours

Ingredients:

- 2 eggs
- 1 pound white fish fillets, skinless, boneless and cut into medium strips
- Black pepper to the taste
- 1 cup almond flour
- ¼ teaspoon paprika
- Cooking spray

Directions:

1. In a bowl, mix the flour with pepper and paprika and stir.
2. Put the eggs in another bowl and whisk them well
3. Dip fish sticks in the egg, dredge in flour mix, arrange them in your slow cooker greased with cooking spray, cover and cook on High for 2 hours.
4. Serve them as an appetizer.

Nutrition Info:

Calories 403, Fat 24.5g, Cholesterol 169mg, Sodium 171mg, Carbohydrate 7.1g, Fiber 3.1g, Sugars 0.6g, Protein 36.6g, Potassium 493mg

Soy Sauce Chicken Wings

Servings: 6

Cooking Time: 3 Hours

Ingredients:

- 3 pounds chicken wings
- 2 and ¼ cups pineapple juice, unsweetened
- 1 teaspoon olive oil
- 3 tablespoons low sodium soy sauce
- 2 tablespoons almond flour
- 2 tablespoons garlic, minced
- 1 tablespoon ginger, minced
- 2 tablespoons 5 spice powder
- A pinch of red pepper flakes, crushed

Directions:

1. Put the pineapple juice in your slow cooker, add the oil, ginger, soy sauce, garlic and flour and whisk really well.
2. Season chicken wings with pepper flakes and 5-spice powder, add them to your slow cooker, cover and cook on High for 3 hours.

3. Transfer chicken wings to a platter, drizzle some of the sauce over them and serve as an appetizer.

Nutrition Info:

Calories 568, Fat 23.2g, Cholesterol 202mg, Sodium 506mg, Carbohydrate 18.4g, Fiber 1.4g, Sugars 11.7g, Protein 68.7g, Potassium 713mg

3-ingredients Shrimp Salad

Servings: 4

Cooking Time: 3 Hours

Ingredients:

- 3 pounds shrimp, peeled and deveined
- 14 ounces canned tomato paste, no-salt-added
- 1 red onion, chopped

Directions:

1. In your slow cooker, mix shrimp with onion and tomato paste, stir, cover and cook on Low for 3 hours.
2. Divide into small bowls and serve.

Nutrition Info:

Calories 497, Fat 6.3g, Cholesterol 716mg, Sodium 928mg, Carbohydrate 26.5g, Fiber 4.7g, Sugars 13.3g, Protein 82.1g, Potassium 1623mg

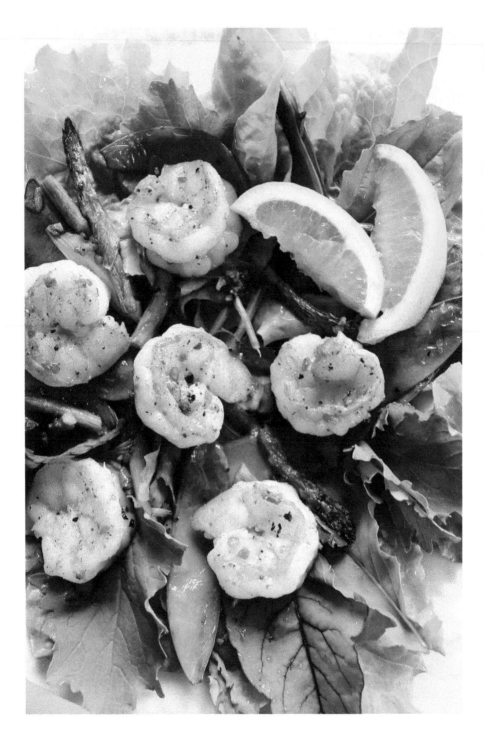

Stevia And Bulgur Salad

Servings: 4

Cooking Time: 8 Hours

Ingredients:

- 2 cups white mushrooms, sliced
- 14 ounces canned kidney beans, no-salt-added, drained
- 14 ounces canned pinto beans, no-salt-added, drained
- 2 cups yellow onion, chopped
- 1 cup low sodium veggie stock
- 1 cup strong coffee
- ¾ cup bulgur, soaked and drained
- ½ cup red bell pepper, chopped
- 2 garlic cloves, minced
- 2 tablespoons stevia
- 2 tablespoons chili powder
- 1 tablespoon cocoa powder
- 1 teaspoon oregano, dried
- 2 teaspoons cumin, ground
- Black pepper to the taste

Directions:

1. In your slow cooker, mix mushrooms with bulgur, onion, bell pepper, stock, garlic, coffee, kidney and pinto beans, stevia, chili powder, cocoa, oregano, cumin and pepper, stir gently, cover and cook on Low for 12 hours.

2. Divide the mix into small bowls and serve cold as an appetizer.

Nutrition Info:

Calories 837, Fat 4.2g, Cholesterol 0mg, Sodium 165mg, Carbohydrate 162g, Fiber 39.1g, Sugars 9.1g, Protein 49.9g, Potassium 3227mg

4-WEEK MEAL PLAN

Week 1

Monday
Breakfast: Tofu Frittata
Lunch: Pork Chops In Beer
Dinner: Stewed Tomatoes

Tuesday
Breakfast: Tapioca
Lunch: Creamy Beef Burgundy
Dinner: Oregano Salad

Wednesday
Breakfast: Fruit Oats
Lunch: Smothered Steak
Dinner: Black Beans With Corn Kernels

Thursday
Breakfast: Grapefruit Mix
Lunch: Pork For Sandwiches
Dinner: Stuffed Acorn Squash

Friday
Breakfast: Berry Yogurt
Lunch: Cranberry Pork Roast
Dinner: Greek Eggplant

Saturday

Breakfast: Soft Pudding

Lunch: Pan-asian Pot Roast

Dinner: Thyme Sweet Potatoes

Sunday

Breakfast: Black Beans Salad

Lunch: Short Ribs

Dinner: Barley Vegetable Soup

Week 2

Monday

Breakfast: Carrot Pudding

Lunch: French Dip

Dinner: Butter Corn

Tuesday

Breakfast: Apple Cake

Lunch: Italian Roast With Vegetables

Dinner: Orange Glazed Carrots

Wednesday

Breakfast: Almond Milk Barley Cereals

Lunch: Honey Mustard Ribs

Dinner: Cinnamon Acorn Squash

Thursday

Breakfast: Cashews Cake

Lunch: Pizza Casserole

Dinner: Glazed Root Vegetables

Friday

Breakfast: Artichoke Frittata

Lunch: Hawaiian Pork Roast

Dinner: Stir Fried Steak, Shiitake And Asparagus

Saturday

Breakfast: Mexican Eggs

Lunch: Apple Cranberry Pork Roast

Dinner: Cilantro Brussel Sprouts

Sunday

Breakfast: Stewed Peach

Lunch: Swiss Steak

Dinner: Italian Zucchini

Week 3

Monday

Breakfast: Lamb Cassoule t

Lunch: Glazed Pork Roast

Dinner: Cilantro Parsnip Chunks

Tuesday

Breakfast: Fruited Tapioca

Lunch: Swiss Steak In Wine Sauce

Dinner: Corn Casserole

Wednesday

Breakfast: Baby Spinach Shrimp Salad

Lunch: Italian Pork Chops

Dinner: Pilaf With Bella Mushrooms

Thursday

Breakfast: Coconut And Fruit Cake

Lunch: Italian Pot Roast

Dinner: Italian Style Yellow Squash

Friday

Breakfast: Apple And Squash Bowls

Lunch: Beef With Horseradish Sauce

Dinner: Stevia Peas With Marjoram

Saturday

Breakfast: Slow Cooker Chocolate Cake

Lunch: Oriental Pot Roast

Dinner: Broccoli Rice Casserole

Sunday

Breakfast: Fish Omelet

Lunch: Barbecued Ribs

Dinner: Italians Style Mushroom Mix

Week 4

Monday
Breakfast: Brown Cake
Lunch: Ham And Scalloped Pota toes
Dinner: Broccoli Casserole

Tuesday
Breakfast: Stevia And Walnuts Cut Oats
Lunch: Pork And Pineapple Roast

Wednesday
Breakfast: Walnut And Cinnamon Oatmeal
Lunch: Barbecued Brisket
Dinner: Dinner: Slow Cooker Lasagna

Thursday
Breakfast: Tender Rosemary Sweet Potatoes
Lunch: Barbecued Short Ribs
Dinner: Brussels Sprouts Casserole

Friday
Breakfast: Orange And Maple Syrup Quinoa
Lunch: Beer-braised Short Ribs
Dinner: Pasta And Mushrooms

Saturday
Breakfast: Vanilla And Nutmeg Oatmeal
Lunch: Lamb Stew
Dinner: Onion Cabbage

Sunday

Breakfast: Pecans Cake

Lunch: Barbecued Ham

Dinner: Cheese Broccoli

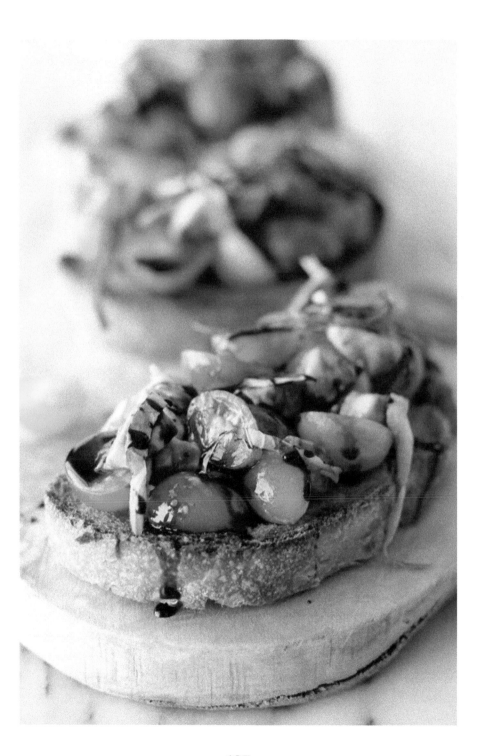